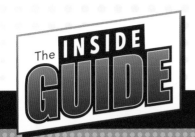

# ROBOTICS

## Robots in
# Medicine

By Ronan Rowell

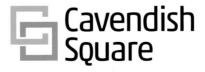

## Cavendish Square

New York

Library of Congress Cataloging-in-Publication Data

Names: Rowell, Ronan, author.
Title: Robots in medicine / Ronan Rowell.
Description: First [edition]. | New York : Cavendish Square Publishing, [2022] | Series: The inside guide: robotics | Includes index.
Identifiers: LCCN 2020025200 | ISBN 9781502660602 (library binding) | ISBN 9781502660589 (paperback) | ISBN 9781502660596 (set) | ISBN 9781502660619 (ebook)
Subjects: LCSH: Robotics in medicine–Juvenile literature. | Robotics–Juvenile literature.
Classification: LCC R857.R63 R69 2022 | DDC 610.285–dc23
LC record available at https://lccn.loc.gov/2020025200

Editor: Caitie McAneney
Copyeditor: Jill Keppeler
Designer: Deanna Paternostro

The photographs in this book are used by permission and through the courtesy of: Cover Zapp2Photo/Shutterstock.com; p. 4 Jaffé/ullstein bild via Getty Images; p. 6 Mikael Sjoberg/Bloomberg via Getty Images; p. 7 (top) Kathryn Scott Osler/The Denver Post via Getty Images; p. 7 (bottom) Khaled Nasraoui/picture alliance via Getty Images; p. 8 Cesar Manso/AFP via Getty Images; p. 9 Francis Demange/Gamma-Rapho via Getty Images; p. 10 Dong Ning/Visual China Group via Getty Images; p. 12 (top) PhotoAlto/Odilon Dimier/PhotoAlto Agency RF Collections/Getty Images; p. 12 (bottom) Mark Harmel/Alamy Stock Photo; p. 13 Thomas Samson/AFP via Getty Images; p. 14 Stocktrek Images/Stocktrek Images/Getty Images; p. 15 Wavebreakmedia/iStock/Getty Images Plus/Getty Images; p. 16 Steve Parsons/Pool/AFP via Getty Images; p. 18 (top) Stan Honda/AFP via Getty Images; p. 18 (bottom) Richard Newstead/The Image Bank/Getty Images; p. 19 Odd Andersen/AFP via Getty Images; p. 20 andresr/E+/Getty Images; p. 21 Casanowe/iStock/Getty Images Plus/Getty Images; p. 22 Imagno/Hulton Archive/Getty Images; p. 24 Craig F. Walker/The Boston Globe via Getty Images; p. 25 (top) Leonard Ortiz/Digital First Media/Orange County Register via Getty Images; p. 25 (bottom) Costfoto/Barcroft Media via Getty Images; p. 26 ullstein bild/Contributor/ullstein bild/Getty Images; p. 27 Manjunath Kiran/AFP via Getty Images; p. 28 (top) Anton Raharjo/Anadolu Agency via Getty Images; p. 28 (bottom) Vachira Vachira/NurPhoto via Getty Images; p. 29 (top) Pete Marovich/Bloomberg via Getty Images; p. 29 (bottom) Mario Tama/Getty Images News/Getty Images.

Some of the images in this book illustrate individuals who are models. The depictions do not imply actual situations or events.

CPSIA compliance information: Batch #CS22CSQ: For further information contact Cavendish Square Publishing LLC, New York, New York, at 1-877-980-4450.

Printed in the United States of America

Find us on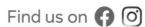

# CONTENTS

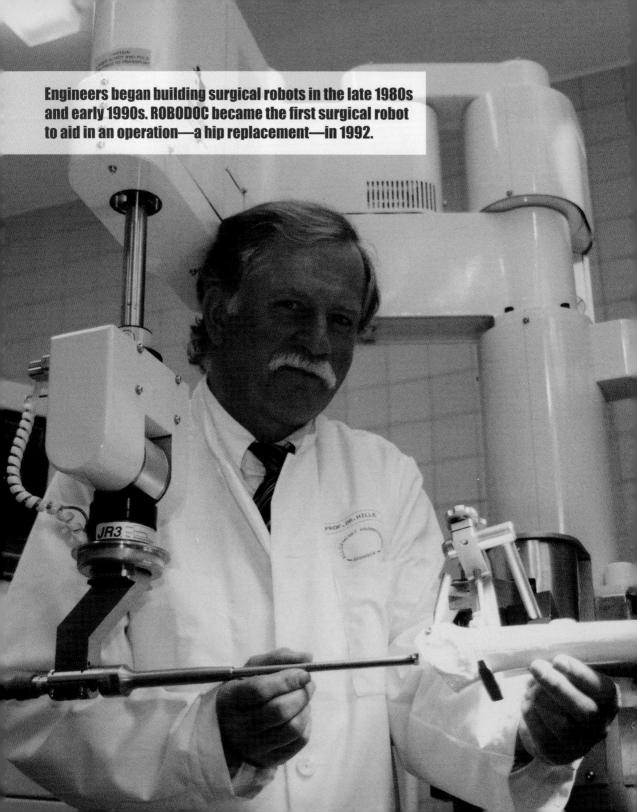

Engineers began building surgical robots in the late 1980s and early 1990s. ROBODOC became the first surgical robot to aid in an operation—a hip replacement—in 1992.

# HELP IN HOSPITALS

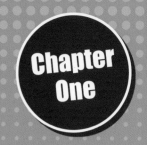

# Chapter One

Robots are more than just high-tech toys. In some cases, they can save lives! Today, robots work alongside medical professionals to treat patients. They can help perform surgeries, produce lifesaving medical **equipment**, and deliver medicine and supplies to hard-to-reach places. Robots can also reduce the risk of spreading sickness. Their hospital help is not only useful, it's necessary.

## Telehealth Teamwork

Have you ever had a telehealth doctor's appointment? Many medical and mental health professionals offer appointments through video chat apps. This is especially important during outbreaks of diseases, such as the COVID-19 **pandemic**, which started in 2019. Telehealth technology allows health-care professionals to talk to patients without coming into physical contact with them.

### Fast Fact

Telepresence is the use of **virtual reality** technology to take part in something from a different place.

Robots can help with telepresence in hospitals. They can move through the halls of hospitals, helping doctors **diagnose** patients from afar when people may be **contagious**. In April 2020, Spot, a robotic dog

# ROBOT REVIEW

Robots come in all sizes and shapes and may have many abilities. While some robots are very large and work in factories producing medical equipment, others are so small they can fit in the human body. However, all robots have the same basic parts. A robot's sensors help it see, hear, and gather information. A robot's controller is like its brain, programmed with information it needs to perform its tasks. Some robots are preprogrammed to perform tasks, while others are controlled remotely, or from a distance. The controller also operates effectors and actuators, a robot's moving parts. Effectors allow robots to perform specific tasks, while actuators are the motors that allow effectors to do their jobs.

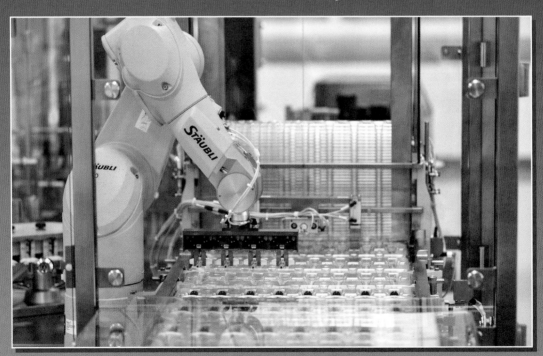

Industrial, or factory, robots such as this one can produce important drugs and medical supplies.

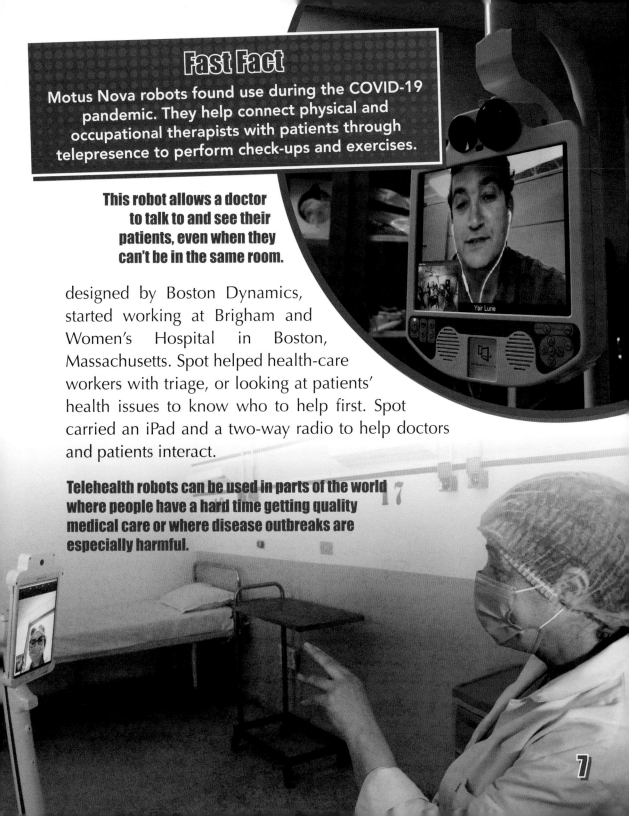

**This robot allows a doctor to talk to and see their patients, even when they can't be in the same room.**

designed by Boston Dynamics, started working at Brigham and Women's Hospital in Boston, Massachusetts. Spot helped health-care workers with triage, or looking at patients' health issues to know who to help first. Spot carried an iPad and a two-way radio to help doctors and patients interact.

**Telehealth robots can be used in parts of the world where people have a hard time getting quality medical care or where disease outbreaks are especially harmful.**

7

# Keep It Clean!

Hospitals are places where people go to get better, but they are also full of harmful germs such as bacteria that can make people sick. Hospital workers and other patients are at risk of catching whatever diseases patients bring into the hospital. Some patients' bodies are busy fighting the illnesses they already have, which makes it harder to fight other illnesses. Also, germs can get into surgical incisions, or cuts. That means that hospitals need to be as clean as possible!

Robots can sanitize, or deep-clean, hospitals. Some robots release a mist of chemicals into the air to disinfect an area, or kill all harmful germs in it. Others use ultraviolet (UV) light to kill germs. This is especially important during disease outbreaks and pandemics. Many hospitals, airports, and public spaces started using UV-disinfecting robots like Xenex and Tru-D during the COVID-19 pandemic.

# Orderly Robots

There's a lot of nonmedical work to be done in a hospital, including making

**This robot uses UV light to sanitize public spaces.**

## Fast Fact

UV-disinfecting robots use "light strikes" to clean a room. Light strikes are intense bursts of UV light—so intense than no one else can be in the room when they're happening!

beds and delivering food to patients. These tasks are usually done by a worker called an orderly, but sometimes it's not safe for humans to do this work because of disease. That's where robots come in.

In 2015, a new hospital in San Francisco, California, started using robot orderlies called TUGs. These slow-moving robots roll through the hospital, delivering food and medicines. They also carry laundry and trash from patients' rooms. Medical waste and bedding used by contagious patients can be harmful to human orderlies, but they're no problem for a TUG. TUGs navigate using the hospital's Wi-Fi signals and use onboard sensors to avoid people and objects. The COVID-19 pandemic saw a sharp increase in the numbers of hospitals that wanted to buy TUGs.

**Mobile robots can be useful in hospital settings. They can travel several miles per day, and they never get tired of working.**

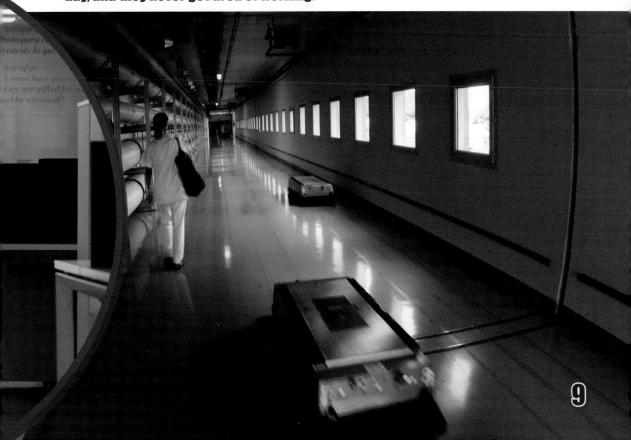

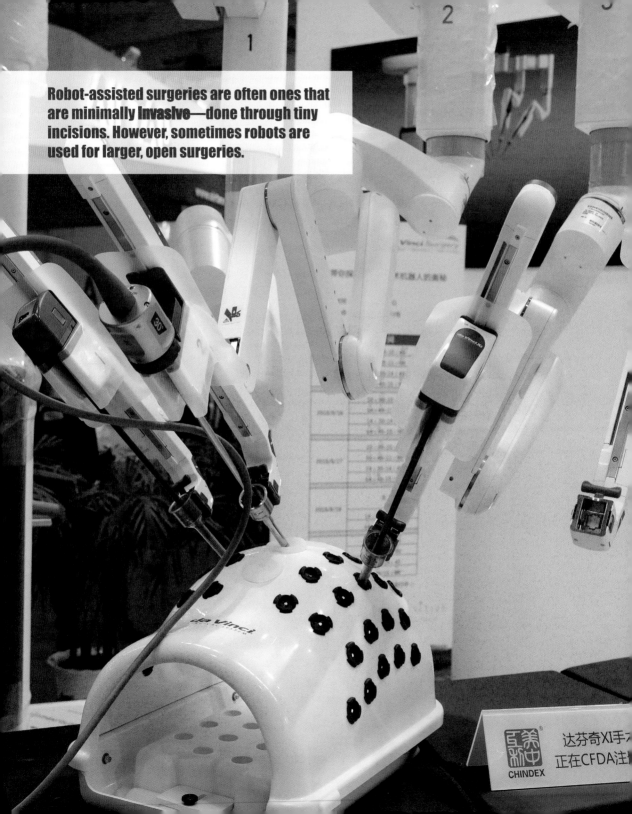

Robot-assisted surgeries are often ones that are minimally **invasive**—done through tiny incisions. However, sometimes robots are used for larger, open surgeries.

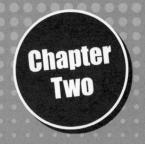

# Chapter Two

# ROBOTIC OPERATIONS

**S**urgeries are major medical **procedures**. Surgeons have to be precise, or exact, in order to fix a part of the human body. Sometimes, doctors even need to **transplant** an organ to keep someone alive. Robots have made lifesaving operations possible, and robotics might be the key to the future of surgery.

## Robot Surgeons

Robots have been used for a long time for their precision and their ability to do the same task over and over without getting tired. That's why they're useful in factories! How can these abilities be used in an operating room?

Robots can't perform surgeries on their own yet—they're still just a tool for surgeons. Most of these robots have an arm with a camera and other arms with surgical instruments. The robot follows the hand movements of the surgeon. A major benefit of surgical robots is that they can perform procedures in a much less invasive way with less harm to the patient. Surgical robots can often perform surgeries with smaller incisions

### Fast Fact

Surgical robots have a camera attached to a long tube called an endoscope. It allows the surgeon to get an up-close, 3-D view of the body part they're operating on.

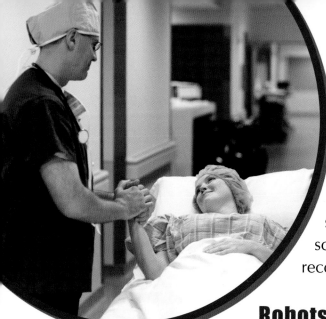

Common robot-assisted surgeries include some heart surgeries and gallbladder removal. Robots may also be used for cutting cancer tissue away from sensitive body parts.

than those made by human surgeons. This can lead to smaller scars, less blood loss, and an easier recovery for a patient.

## Robots at Work Today

Minimally invasive robotic surgery began in the 1980s, with the help of the PUMA 560 surgical arm. The U.S. Army was interested in robotic technology to treat wounded soldiers from a distance. It helped develop AESOP (Automated Endoscopic System for Optimal Positioning), the first robotic surgical system approved by the U.S. Food and Drug Administration (FDA). AESOP could provide real-time video of the area the

Robots are especially useful in laparoscopic procedures, which are when a doctor looks into a person's abdomen with a special scope.

## Fast Fact

The ZEUS surgical system used AESOP technology. It was once a rival to the da Vinci robotic surgery system, but it's no longer used.

# Discover the da Vinci Surgical System

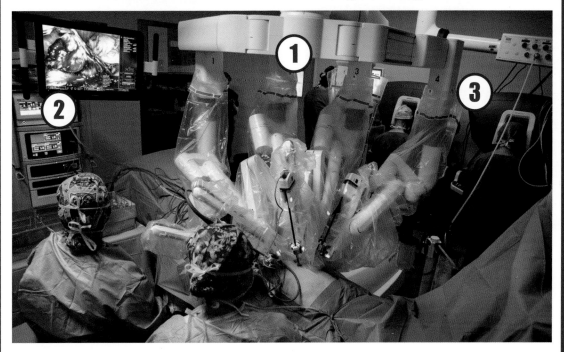

## 1. Patient Cart
- placed over the patient for operation
- holds camera and surgical instruments on arms
- arms controlled by the surgeon from the console

## 2. Vision Cart
- 3-D vision system
- helps doctor see the surgical area as they work

## 3. Surgeon Console
- surgeon sits at this console and their motions control the instruments on the patient cart
- surgeon looks to the vision cart for information that directs their actions

surgeon was operating on. The doctor would give voice commands to the robot, which could move a robotic arm.

In 2000, the da Vinci surgical system was approved by the FDA for general laparoscopic operations. This system is still used today. The system usually involves three robotic arms. Two of the arms respond to the surgeon's left and right arm movements, and one has a camera. A surgeon uses a separate console, or control system, to guide the arms during surgery.

Usually, surgeons are nearby for this kind of robot-assisted surgery. However, in 2019, a surgeon in India performed a robot-assisted heart surgery from 20 miles (32.2 kilometers) away. This may be the beginning of more long-distance robotic surgery, which can save the lives of people who live in faraway areas or soldiers in war zones.

## Nanorobots of the Future!

Engineers and scientists are working on the surgical robots of the future—and some of these robots are tiny! Microrobotics and nanorobotics are branches of robotics that deal with very small robots. Insect-sized microrobots or even cell-sized nanorobots may one day crawl or swim through the human body to treat patients.

**Fast Fact**

Cancer researchers are trying to develop nanorobots that target cancerous cells without harming healthy tissue.

Today, an infection might be treated with weeks of antibiotics, but in the future, nanorobots may be able to get rid of harmful germs inside a patient in minutes. These microscopic robots could even perform surgery at the cellular level by removing or repairing diseased and damaged cells. They could also bring medicine to a specific part of the body. Researchers have already tested nanorobots to fight cancerous cells in mice.

Someday, nanorobots may swim through a person's bloodstream to repair damaged blood cells.

# SMART PILLS AND NANOTECHNOLOGY TODAY

"Smart pills" are a kind of nanotechnology that people can swallow. They contain sensors and cameras. In 2019, scientists developed the Sonopill, a device that, once swallowed, moves through the body and captures images of the intestines. In the past, scientists were unable to keep a pill where it was supposed to take a picture. However, a magnet inside the Sonopill is drawn to a robotic arm hovering over the correct spot on the patient's body. Pills like this could help check for diseases of the gut, including cancer. In the future, nanorobot pills may take direct action in treating diseases through magnetic microsurgery.

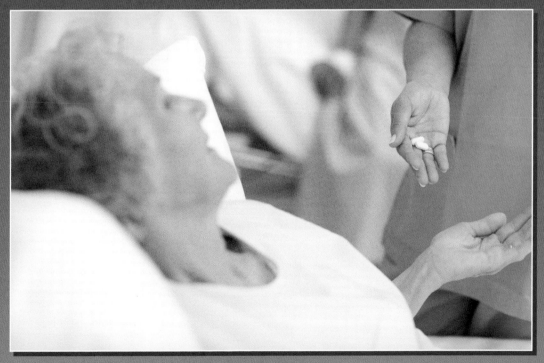

In the future, learning what's wrong with your body when you're ill might be as easy as taking a smart pill.

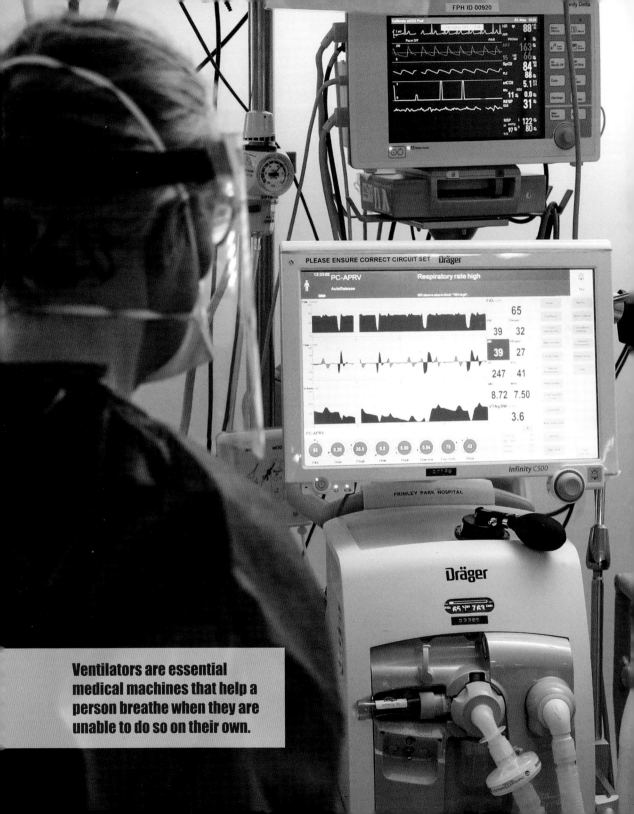

Ventilators are essential medical machines that help a person breathe when they are unable to do so on their own.

# MEDICINE MADE EASIER

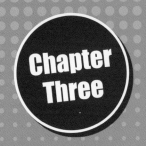
**M**edicine can save lives—and robots can help! From producing important medicines and medical devices in factories to delivering **vaccines** around the world, robots are at the forefront of today's medical production and distribution systems.

## Making Medicine

Industrial robots can be masters of medical production. In factories and warehouses, robots can pick up, assemble, and pack products. This includes medicines as well as important items such as ventilators and personal protective equipment (PPE). In early 2020, as the COVID-19 pandemic first hit the United States, the U.S. government and private companies had to ramp up production of ventilators and PPE, which was a job for industrial robots.

### Fast Fact

In April 2020, Boyce Technologies, which usually produces electronics and computers, repurposed its robot production line and installed a new robot to help make 300 ventilators a day for COVID-19 patients.

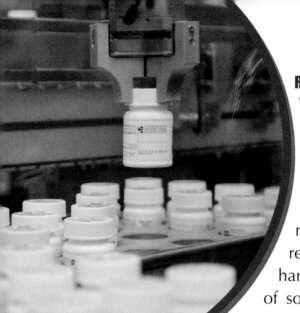

**Robots are often used to fill bottles with the correct number of pills that patients need.**

When it comes to dispensing, or giving, medicine to patients, precision is important. Too little medicine and the patient may not recover, but too much medicine might harm or kill them. Robots are capable of sorting and dispensing different pills. Human pharmacists, or people who give medicine, are still needed to look at each **prescription** as well as clean, refill, and program the system. When robots and humans work together, medicine and supplies can be made and dispensed successfully.

## Lifesaving Deliveries

Some people live or work in hard-to-reach places. Some become stuck in disaster zones following a natural disaster or war. Getting medicines to these people can be a matter of life and death.

Drones can deliver medication, food, and water to people in hard-to-reach places. In 2016, a drone company called Zipline partnered with Rwanda's government to use its drones to deliver medical equipment in the African country. It was the world's first

**Flying robots are sometimes called drones or unmanned aerial vehicles (UAVs).**

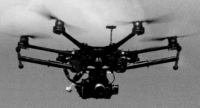

# DELIVERIES OF THE FUTURE!

In the future, drones could deliver medicines and medical equipment to people in their homes. That way, people wouldn't have to go to the hospital or pharmacy to obtain their prescriptions. Drones could deliver necessary blood to rural hospitals and could collect blood samples for health labs. Pandemics and outbreaks, such as the COVID-19 pandemic, can lead to great robotic **innovation**, especially in terms of drone delivery. Robots can ensure less contact between people, which could help stop the spread of disease. In fact, drones have delivered COVID test kits to rural areas around the world.

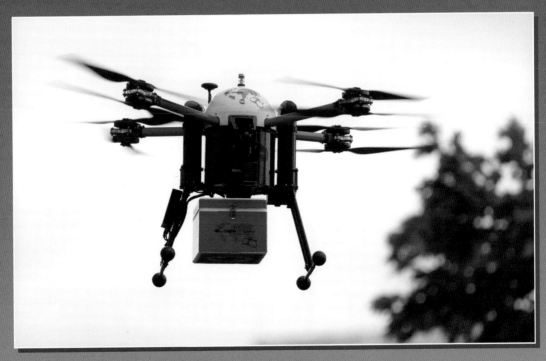

This drone was built for medical deliveries.

national drone delivery program. Soon, the company started sending blood and vaccines to Ghana by drone. When COVID-19 hit the United States, Zipline drones delivered PPE and medical equipment to hospitals in North Carolina.

## Movement Medicine

Sometimes, movement is good medicine! People who are recovering from surgery, illness, or injury often need physical therapy to strengthen their muscles and regain movement.

Robots can help patients move and strengthen their muscles. For example, a robot might help a person gradually work to move their arm after it's injured in an accident.

Robots can also help people who have suffered from neurological (brain) injuries like strokes by helping them relearn how

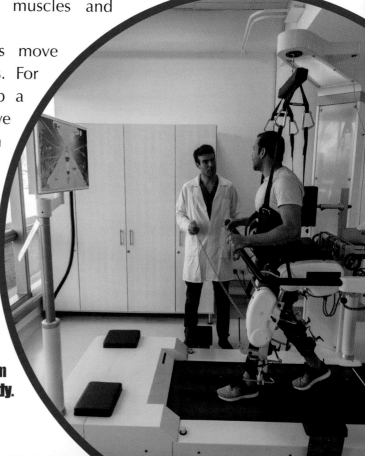

Physical therapists help people strengthen and use their bodies after injury or illness. Robots can help them do their job more efficiently.

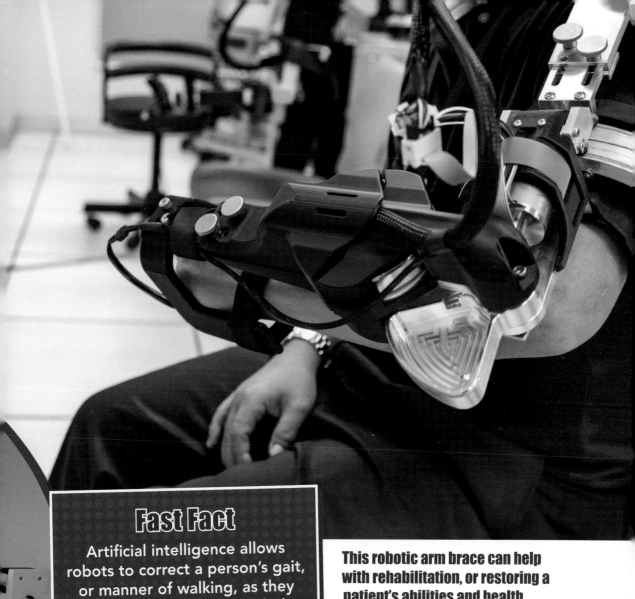

**This robotic arm brace can help with rehabilitation, or restoring a patient's abilities and health.**

to move certain body parts. A robotic harness can be used to physically guide and support people as they build up their strength and **coordination**. This can help people learn to walk again.

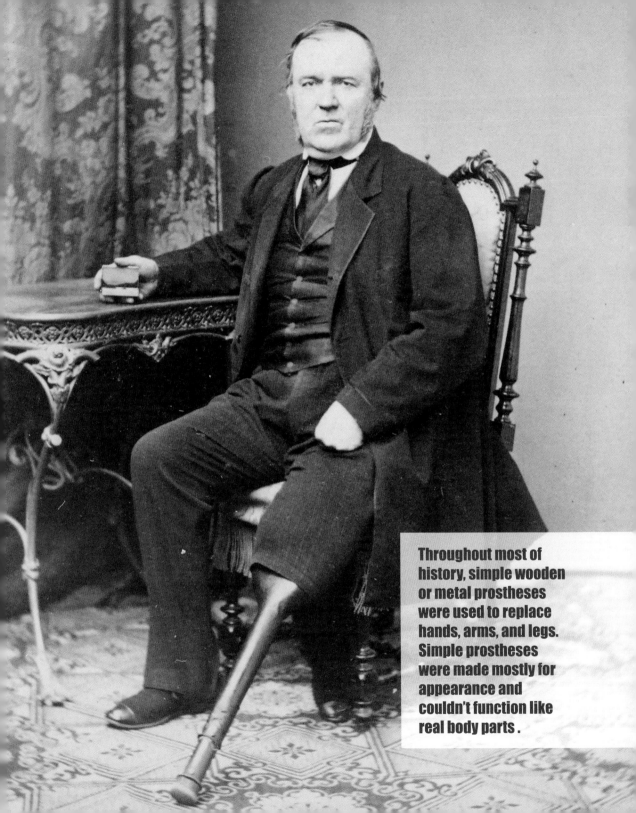

Throughout most of history, simple wooden or metal prostheses were used to replace hands, arms, and legs. Simple prostheses were made mostly for appearance and couldn't function like real body parts .

# A BIONIC FUTURE

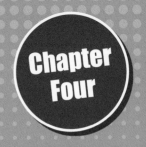
**R**obots and humans work together all the time now, but will they ever combine into bionic people? "Bionic" means having artificial, usually electronic, body parts, and a bionic human is sometimes called a cyborg—especially in science fiction. Thanks to advances in robotics, bionic technology is helping to reshape the future of medicine.

## Practical Prosthetics

For **amputees** and people born without limbs, performing everyday tasks sometimes depends on prostheses. Prostheses are artificial devices used to replace missing body parts.

The BiOM prosthesis by iWalk is a close copy of a functioning human leg, ankle, and foot. The i-Limb robotic hand was the first commercially available advanced prosthetic hand, with fingers that could move individually like those on a real hand.

### Fast Fact

Lost limbs are common injuries in modern wars because of IEDs (improvised explosive devices). Veterans who've lost limbs are in need of advanced prostheses, and robotics is one answer to this problem.

The LUKE prosthetic arm was named after Luke Skywalker from *Star Wars*. It's been in development for about 15 years.

Advanced prostheses such as the iWalk BiOM and i-Limb use electrical signals from the surrounding muscles and nervous system. However, these robotic systems sometimes have electrical signal issues, can be bulky, and don't allow for a sense of touch. New technology aims to fix some of these problems.

In 2019, the LUKE prosthetic arm gave users a sense of touch by linking the robotic arm to a user's nerves. In 2020, scientists developed a way to implant muscle tissue in amputees to help them better communicate nerve signals with a LUKE prosthetic arm. They could move the arm with their mind—a major robotics breakthrough.

## Exciting Exoskeletons

For people living with paralysis, or the inability to move part of their body, everyday activities can be very difficult. Some people are unable to walk because of paralysis, and robotic suits called exoskeletons could help them regain movement.

Exoskeletons are a type of wearable robot that can help

### Fast Fact

As many as 1 in 50 people in the United States have some form of paralysis. Paralysis can happen because of stroke, spinal cord injury, or neurological disorders.

**Exoskeletons like the ReWalk can give people who are paralyzed the ability to walk upright again.**

people with paralysis walk again. They can be used every day, like a wheelchair, or as a temporary physical therapy tool. Exoskeletons can help stroke survivors strengthen weakened muscles and relearn how to move certain body parts. Some hospitals have a patient wear an exoskeleton and walk on a treadmill to strengthen their muscles.

In 2011, ReWalk became the first exoskeleton cleared by the FDA for personal use in the United States. Users can walk, turn, and stand upright while wearing the suit, which could give new abilities to people with paralysis.

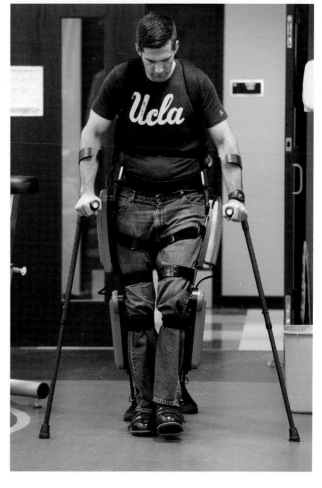

## Hope for Healing

Robotics has had a huge impact on medical care, especially in the past few decades. Today, robots assist during

**Global health issues like COVID-19 challenge engineers to think of new robotic technologies to solve problems— like this "virus-killing" tank.**

# INTRODUCING...CYBORGS?

In 2011, Japanese robotics company Cyberdyne introduced what it calls the world's first cyborg-type robot. HAL, which stands for Hybrid Assistive Limb, is intended to bring together humans and robotic technology to help people regain their ability to walk. The robot uses sensors on the skin that pick up electrical signals from the user's body to direct the robot to move. In 2017, the FDA cleared HAL for use in the United States in medical settings. What sets HAL apart from ReWalk and other wearable robots is that it has a different goal—not to assist a user forever, but to help them eventually walk on their own without it.

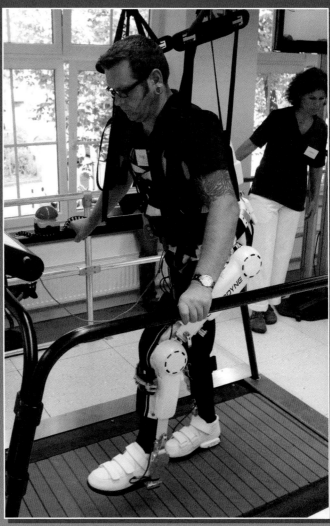

Like other rehabilitation and recovery robots, the HAL exoskeleton helps a person train to walk again.

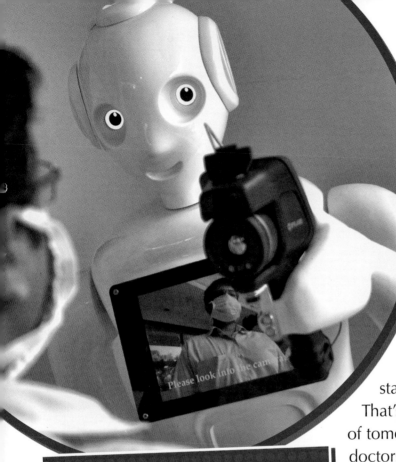

Robots like this one are already being used to take temperatures at hospitals. What else could robots do in the future?

surgical procedures, dispense medicine, and keep hospitals clean. They can help people recover from injuries and help stop the spread of illnesses.

Will a hospital ever be staffed completely by robots? That's unlikely, but the hospitals of tomorrow will probably feature doctors and nurses working alongside robots and robot orderlies. Nanorobots could be used to repair and replace damaged cells. Robotic prostheses and exoskeletons could function just like natural body parts. New technology is being developed every year! Robots provide hope for a future in which people—no matter where they live or what illness or disability they might have—can live a full and healthy life.

**Fast Fact**

Every year, an event called the Hamlyn Symposium on Medical Robotics takes place in London, UK, to bring together leading minds in medicine and robotics and look to the future of medical robots.

# THINK ABOUT IT!

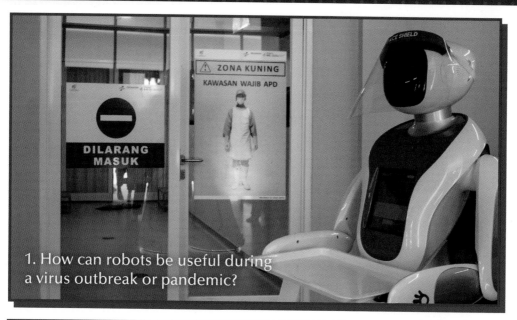

1. How can robots be useful during a virus outbreak or pandemic?

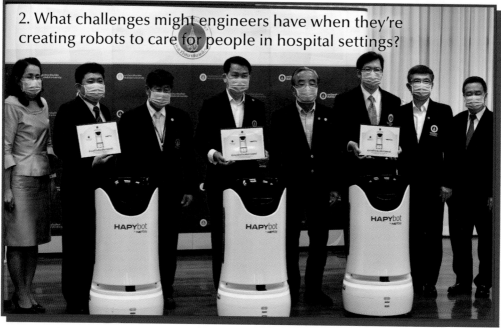

2. What challenges might engineers have when they're creating robots to care for people in hospital settings?

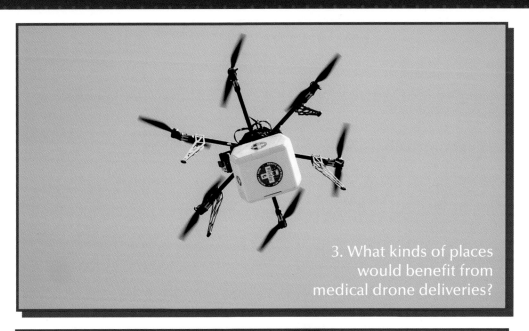

3. What kinds of places would benefit from medical drone deliveries?

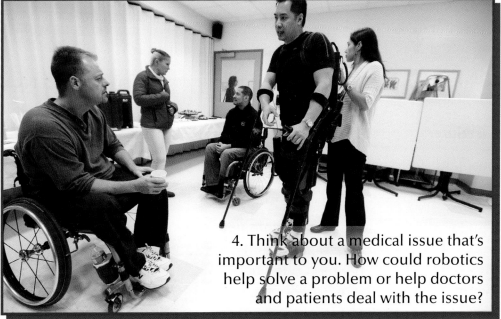

4. Think about a medical issue that's important to you. How could robotics help solve a problem or help doctors and patients deal with the issue?

# GLOSSARY

**amputee:** One who has had a limb removed.

**contagious:** Able to spread infection or disease from one being to another.

**coordination:** Skillful and balanced body movements.

**diagnose:** To recognize a disease by signs and symptoms.

**efficiently:** Having to do with the most effective or purposeful way of doing something.

**equipment:** Tools, clothing, and other items needed for a job.

**innovation:** A new invention or a new way of doing things.

**invasive:** Involving entry into the living body.

**pandemic:** An outbreak of disease that occurs over a wide geographic area and affects a great proportion of the population.

**prescription:** A written direction, often by a doctor, for use of treatments such as medicine.

**procedure:** An operation or other medical treatment.

**transplant:** To transfer a body part from one part or individual to another.

**vaccine:** A shot that keeps a person from getting a certain sickness.

**virtual reality:** An artificial environment which is experienced through sensory effects (such as sights and sounds) provided by a computer and in which one's actions partially determine what happens in the environment.

# FIND OUT MORE

## Books

Higgins, Nadia. *Medical Robots*. Mankato, MN: Amicus Ink, 2018.

Hulick, Kathryn and Michael Yip. *Medical Robots*. Minneapolis, MN: Abdo Publishing, 2019.

Noll, Elizabeth. *Medical Robots*. Minneapolis, MN: Bellwether Media, 2018.

## Websites

### All About Robotics
*easyscienceforkids.com/all-about-robotics/*
Robotics is reshaping our world! Learn more about how robots are used in different fields on this website.

### Nanotechnology
*www.brainpop.com/technology/scienceandindustry/nanotechnology/*
This BrainPop lesson will introduce you to the exciting world of nanotechnology.

### Robot Facts for Kids
*kids.kiddle.co/Robot*
This website is full of fun facts about robots.

# INDEX